CATAPLEXY

LIFESTYLE TREATMENTS FOR CATAPLEXY

DR. J. SIMON

Contents

INTRODUCTION

One interesting but difficult side effect of narcolepsy is cataplexy. It resembles a turn in the narcoleptic tale. Cataplexy is essentially characterized by an abrupt loss of muscle tone brought on by intense feelings like laughter, excitement, or even rage. Imagine this: during a hilarious moment, your muscles choose to voluntarily relax rather than simply laughing it off. It's similar to a brief system failure that renders you immobile.

Each experiences cataplexy to a different degree. While some may have more severe episodes where they completely collapse, others may only experience mild muscle weakness. Although it's not harmful in and of itself, it can certainly make things more difficult in daily life.

It's interesting to note that narcolepsy, a neurological condition marked by excessive daytime sleepiness and a propensity to fall asleep unexpectedly, is frequently associated with cataplexy. They act as accomplices in crime, adding an element of unpredictability to the lives of those they interact with.

CHAPTER ONE

What Cataplexy Is Definition

A sudden and transient loss of muscle tone or strength is known as cataplexy, a neurological phenomenon that is typically brought on by intense emotions like stress, laughter, or excitement. It can occur on its own, but it is most frequently linked to the sleep disorder narcolepsy. A person may have a variety of symptoms during a cataplectic episode, ranging from slight muscle weakness to total muscle paralysis, which may result in a transient incapacity to move or speak. Although cataplexy is generally not harmful, it can have a major effect on activities and daily life.

Comprehending Cataplexy

Gaining insight into cataplexy necessitates exploring the complex realm of the nervous system. Narcolepsy and cataplexy are closely related conditions that highlight the delicate neurotransmitter balance in the brain.

Cataplexy can be thought of as a malfunction in the system. Imagine that your brain misinterprets feelings as telling you to press the button for muscular relaxation. Strong emotions, especially happy ones like laughter, cause the brain to send conflicting signals that cause a sudden loss of muscle control. It feels like your body abruptly deviates into a momentary paralysis.

Hypocretin is the main neurotransmitter in this neuronal drama; it controls both REM sleep and wakefulness. Hypocretin deficiency frequently occurs in narcoleptics and cataplexy sufferers, which throws off the regular checks and balances of the sleep-wake cycle.

Thus, cataplexy can be understood as a special example of the intricate relationship that exists between emotions, neurotransmitters, and the brain's regulation of muscular activity. Knowing about it helps to illuminate the complex dance of chemistry and signals that occurs within the human body, as well as the difficulties that those who experience it face.

Basis Neurological

The neurotransmitter hypocretin, also referred to as orexin, is deficient in cataplexy, which is the neurological basis of the condition. Maintaining muscle tone and controlling the sleep-wake cycle are two important functions of hypocretin.

The production of hypocretin is frequently significantly reduced in people with cataplexy, mainly as a result of the death of neurons that generate this neurotransmitter. Particularly noticeable is this loss of neurons that produce hypocretin in the hypothalamus, a part of the brain in charge of many physiological processes, including sleep regulation.

A hormone called hypocretin helps to promote wakefulness and prevent REM (rapid eye movement) sleep. Cataplexy is a condition where there is a hypocretin shortage, which interferes with the regular cycles of wakefulness and sleep.

A spike in emotions during emotional triggers, like laughter or excitement, can cause a sudden inhibition of motor neurons. The brain would normally maintain muscle tone in people without cataplexy, but in people with cataplexy, a hypocretin deficiency permits this inhibition to result in a transient loss of muscle control.

Therefore, the fundamental neurological cause of cataplexy is the dysregulation of hypocretin, which upsets the delicate balance that permits smooth wakefulness and sleep transitions and results in the unusual phenomenon of abrupt paralysis or weakness of the muscles during emotional experiences.

Orexin's function

One of the main factors contributing to cataplexy is orexin, sometimes referred to as hypocretin. The hypothalamus, a part of the brain essential for controlling a number of physiological processes, including wakefulness and sleep, is where these neurotransmitters are made.

Orexin's main job is to control the sleep-wake cycle and encourage wakefulness. It helps keep muscles taut while awake and keeps rapid eye movement (REM) sleep from invading awake periods. When neurons that produce the neurotransmitter orexin are lost, people who have cataplexy have insufficient amounts of this neurotransmitter.

Cataplexy usually occurs during emotional experiences, such as laughter or excitement, when there is a spike in emotions. The normal inhibitory control over motor neurons weakens in people deficient in orexin. Cataplexy is characterized by a sudden loss of muscle control as a result of disruptions to the signals that normally maintain muscle tone.

Hence, orexin maintains equilibrium during the complex dance between wakefulness and sleep. When levels are low, especially during periods of intense emotion, it can lead to cataplexy, which is characterized by a transient, frequently unanticipated loss of muscle tone or paralysis. Gaining knowledge about orexin's function can help one better understand the neurobiology of cataplexy and how it relates to narcolepsy.

Brain Areas Concerned

A number of brain regions are involved in cataplexy, but the hypothalamus and its neurotransmitter orexin are particularly prominent. The main brain regions involved are broken down as follows:

Hypothalamus: This brain region plays a major role in controlling a number of physiological processes, such as wakefulness and sleep. The neurons that generate orexin/hypocretin, a neurotransmitter essential for preserving muscle tone and wakefulness, are housed there. The loss of these neurons in the hypothalamus causes a deficiency of orexin in people with cataplexy.

The brain's deep-seated, almond-shaped amygdala is largely responsible for processing emotions. Amygdala activity spikes during emotional experiences like excitement or laughter. This increased emotional activity may be the catalyst for the loss of muscular control in cataplexy.

Brainstem: The medulla and pons, in particular, are parts of the brainstem that are involved in controlling muscle tone and motor coordination. Cataplexy is characterized by muscle weakness or paralysis, which can be attributed to disruptions in these areas.

Frontal Cortex: Higher cognitive functions and motor control are linked to the frontal cortex. Even though it might not be the main location of cataplectic activity, its interactions with other regions help make symptoms appear.

Deciphering the complex intercommunication between these brain regions is necessary to comprehend cataplexy. The distinct phenomenon of sudden and transient loss of muscle tone in people with cataplexy is caused by a deficiency of orexin in the hypothalamus, emotional triggers, and disturbances in motor control areas.

Causes of Cataplexy

Strong emotions are typically linked to the specific triggers that cause cataplexy. The following are the most typical emotional triggers for cataplexy:

Laughter: Laughing is one of the most well-known cataplexy triggers. An episode of cataplectic seizures is more likely to occur when laughter is more intense.

Excitement: Cataplexy can also be brought on by extreme excitement or happy feelings. This could have to do with happy occasions, startling news, or any other emotionally charged circumstance.

Stress: Cataplexy can be triggered by negative emotions, especially stress or anxiety. Episodes may result from high-stress circumstances or unexpected anxiety-inducing events.

Anger: Some people experience cataplexy when they experience intense feelings of anger or frustration. Anger's intense emotional content can cause muscular weakness and upset the neurotransmitter balance.

It's crucial to remember that each person with cataplexy will respond differently to these triggers, and that not everyone will experience episodes in response to the same emotions. Furthermore, some people might not have clear triggers, and cataplexy can happen on its own. In order to manage and cope with cataplexy, it can be helpful to recognize and understand one's own triggers.

The signs and symptoms of cataplexy can vary widely, from slight muscle weakness to total paralysis. The following are the main signs and symptoms of cataplexy:

Muscle Weakness: The most typical symptom is an abrupt loss of muscle tone, which makes the muscles weak. This can range in severity from mild facial muscle sagging to more noticeable weakness in larger muscle groups.

Facial Drooping: Cataplexy frequently affects the facial muscles, causing slurred speech or facial drooping. It's possible that the person has trouble maintaining facial expressions or speaking clearly.

Knee Buckling: Weakness in the knees can make some people's knees buckle or give way. This may cause a brief incapacity to walk or stand.

Total Collapse: In more extreme circumstances, cataplexy may result in a total loss of muscle control, which would cause the person to collapse. Even though they are completely conscious, they might become momentarily immobile.

Episode Length: Catalectic episodes usually have a short duration, ranging from a few seconds to several minutes. Muscle tone gradually returns to normal after the emotional trigger passes.

Triggers and Emotional Context: Strong emotions, particularly happy ones like joy or laughter, are frequently what set off cataplexy. Stress, rage, or other strong emotions can also cause it to happen.

Normal Consciousness: It's significant to note that people who experience cataplexy maintain full consciousness throughout the episodes. There is no loss of consciousness, in contrast to fainting or seizures.

It is important for those who are experiencing cataplexy as well as those around them to be aware of the variety of symptoms linked to the condition. It draws attention to the special way that emotions, the neurological system, and muscular control interact in this fascinating neurological phenomenon.

CHAPTER TWO

Length and Intensity

There is a large range in the length and intensity of cataplexy in different people. The following are some broad observations:

Time: Catapaclectic episodes usually last anywhere from a few seconds to a few minutes. Factors like the strength of the emotional trigger and individual variations in the nervous system's response can affect how long it lasts.

Severity: Cataplexy can also range in severity. In less severe instances, people might feel a little weakness in their face muscles or a brief moment of knee buckling. In more extreme cases, there might be a total loss of muscle control, which could result in a transient collapse.

Individual Variation: The experience of cataplexy varies from person to person. While some people may only have mild, sporadic episodes, others may have more severe, frequent episodes.

Cataplexy Severity is Influenced by Triggers: The emotional trigger affects how severe the condition becomes. Intense laughter or excitement, for instance, can cause more prominent episodes than circumstances involving softer emotional stimuli.

Effect on Daily Life: Depending on the frequency and intensity of episodes, cataplexy can have varying effects on daily life. While some people may find it easier to cope and manage in some circumstances, others may find it more difficult.

Working closely with healthcare professionals to develop strategies for managing and minimizing the impact of cataplexy on daily life is crucial for individuals affected by the condition. Cataplexy and its related symptoms can be effectively managed with a comprehensive approach that includes lifestyle modifications and medication.

Effects on Day-to-Day Living

A person's everyday life can be greatly affected by cataplexy, affecting many facets of their routine and social interactions. The following are some ways that living with cataplexy may be impacted:

Social Interactions: People who are afraid of causing cataplexy may restrict their emotional expression or steer clear of particular social situations. Social interactions and relationships may be impacted by this.

Workplace Difficulties: Depending on the intensity and frequency of their cataplectic episodes, people may have difficulties at their jobs. Employment involving a lot of physical coordination or high levels of emotional stress may be especially impacted.

Safety concerns: A sudden loss of muscle control can be dangerous, particularly when driving or using heavy machinery is involved. It might be essential to make lifestyle changes and safety precautions.

Emotional Well-Being: Stress and anxiety can be exacerbated by cataplexy's unpredictable nature. Managing the anxiety of having episodes in front of others or at significant occasions can impact one's emotional health in general.

Sleep Disruption: Narcolepsy and cataplexy are frequently linked conditions that can cause sleep disturbances. Oversleeping during the day and the need for naps to cope with exhaustion can affect day-to-day functioning.

Treatment considerations: Medication, lifestyle modifications, and continuous medical supervision may all be necessary to manage cataplexy. For those who have cataplexy, juggling treatment options and possible side effects can be a daily struggle.

Educational Implications: Academic performance and extracurricular activity participation may be negatively impacted by cataplexy in students. It's possible that administrators and teachers need to be supportive and knowledgeable.

Many people with cataplexy manage to adapt and lead happy lives in spite of these obstacles. To minimize the impact of cataplexy on daily life, it is imperative to maintain open communication with healthcare professionals, enlist the support of friends and family, and take a proactive approach to managing triggers and symptoms.

Differential diagnosis and diagnosis

A comprehensive assessment by medical professionals usually neurologists or sleep specialists is required to diagnose cataplexy. Below is a summary of the diagnostic procedure along with some differential diagnosis considerations:

1. Clinical Assessment:

Medical History: Physicians will take a thorough medical history, covering the patient's sleep habits, level of alertness during the day, and any instances of abrupt muscle weakness or collapse.

Family History: Since there is a genetic component to narcolepsy and cataplexy, a family history may be significant.

2. Research on Sleep:

Polysomnography (PSG): This is an overnight sleep study that evaluates sleep patterns and finds anomalies by monitoring a number of physiological parameters, such as heart rate, muscle activity, brain activity, and eye movement.

The Multiple Sleep Latency Test (MSLT) is a daytime assessment that gauges how long it takes an individual to nod off for scheduled naps. During these naps, people with narcolepsy frequently exhibit a rapid onset of REM sleep.

3. Assessment of Cataplexy:

Clinical History: In-depth questioning regarding bouts of paralysis or muscle weakness brought on by feelings like excitement or laughter.

Observation: If it is feasible, direct observation of cataplectic episodes can help with the diagnosis.

Diagnostic Differentiation:

Cataplexy-like symptoms can be present in a number of conditions, so it's important to rule out other causes. These could consist of:

Disorders of the Seizures: Some seizures resemble cataplexy. Monitoring of the electroencephalogram, or EEG, can assist in distinguishing between seizures and cataplexy.

Seizures known as psychogenic nonepileptic seizures (PNES) can mimic cataplexy and have a psychological cause. It is helpful to differentiate between PNES and cataplexy using video EEG monitoring.

Movement Disorders: Cataplexy and certain movement disorders, such as catatonia, may share characteristics.

Syncope: Episodes of fainting can occasionally be confused with cataplexy. Monitoring heart rate and blood pressure during an episode may be part of the evaluation process.

Neurological Disorders: A thorough neurological examination is required, as some neurological conditions may present with muscle weakness.

Psychiatric Conditions: Cataplexy-like symptoms can be present in conditions like anxiety or panic attacks.

Creating a suitable treatment plan requires an accurate diagnosis. Working together with medical professionals and doing a comprehensive evaluation are essential to distinguishing cataplexy from other disorders that share its symptoms.

Clinical Evaluation

Healthcare practitioners conduct a thorough examination as part of the clinical assessment of cataplexy in order to learn more about the patient's symptoms, medical history, and possible triggers. An outline of the clinical assessment procedure is provided below:

1. Background Information on Health:

Sleep Patterns: Asking detailed questions concerning the patient's sleeping patterns, including the quantity and quality of their nocturnal slumber as well as any problems with excessive daytime sleepiness.

Evaluate the degree of vigilance during the day and any excessive drowsiness during the day, as this is frequently linked to narcolepsy.

Episodes of Weakness: a thorough examination of instances of abrupt paralysis or weakness of the muscles, with an emphasis on pinpointing triggers like stress, excitement, humor, or other feelings.

2. Family Background:

Since there is a genetic component to both narcolepsy and cataplexy, it is advisable to find out if there is a family history of these conditions.

3. Physical Evaluation:

A comprehensive neurological examination is performed to evaluate coordination, reflexes, and motor function.

4. Research on Sleep:

Polysomnography (PSG): An overnight sleep study used to track the heart rate, muscles, brain activity, and eye movement among other physiological parameters during sleep.

The Multiple Sleep Latency Test (MSLT) is a daytime test that involves taking several naps to gauge how quickly a person falls asleep and whether they are experiencing rapid eye movement (REM) sleep.

5. Monitoring Cataplectic Episodes

Clinical History: In-depth inquiry concerning the features of cataplectic episodes, including the predisposing conditions and the length of the episodes.

Video Documentation: When feasible, videotape episodes of cataplectic seizures to obtain important visual data for diagnosis.

6. Diagnostic Differentiation:

Exclusion of Other Conditions: Taking into account and eliminating other medical conditions, such as movement disorders, seizure disorders, or psychiatric conditions, that could mimic cataplexy.

The clinical assessment is a cooperative process that entails open communication and in-depth symptom investigation between the patient and the healthcare professional. The objective is to collect data that will help with precise diagnosis and suitable treatment plan formulation for cataplexy and any associated sleep disorders.

Distinguishing Cataplexy from Other Conditions

Distinguishing cataplexy from other conditions involves a careful consideration of symptoms, triggers, and diagnostic tests. Here are key points to help differentiate cataplexy from other conditions:

1. Emotional Triggers:

Cataplexy: Sudden muscle weakness or paralysis triggered by strong positive emotions such as laughter, excitement, or joy is a hallmark of cataplexy.

Seizures: While seizures can also cause muscle weakness or loss of consciousness, they are not typically triggered by emotions. EEG monitoring can help differentiate between cataplexy and seizures.

Psychogenic Nonepileptic Seizures (PNES): Similar to seizures, PNES are psychological in origin but may lack the specific emotional triggers seen in cataplexy.

2. Sleep Patterns and Narcolepsy:

Cataplexy: Often occurs in individuals with narcolepsy, a condition characterized by excessive daytime sleepiness, fragmented nighttime sleep, and other sleep-related symptoms.

Sleep Disorders: Conditions like sleep paralysis, hypnagogic hallucinations, or other parasomnias may have distinct features that help differentiate them from cataplexy.

3. Video Documentation:

Cataplexy: Video recording of cataplectic episodes, if available, can provide valuable visual information about the nature and characteristics of the episodes.

Other Conditions: Video documentation can aid in distinguishing cataplexy from conditions like psychogenic nonepileptic seizures, where movements may appear more purposeful.

4. Neurological Examination:

Cataplexy: Thorough neurological examination may reveal no abnormalities between episodes, as cataplexy is primarily triggered by emotions.

Movement Disorders: Other movement disorders may present with persistent neurological signs and symptoms even in the absence of emotional triggers.

5. Research on Sleep:

Cataplexy: Polysomnography (PSG) and Multiple Sleep Latency Test (MSLT) can help diagnose narcolepsy and cataplexy by assessing sleep architecture and daytime sleep tendencies.

Other Sleep Disorders: Specific sleep study findings can help identify and differentiate cataplexy from other sleep disorders.

Accurate diagnosis often involves collaboration between neurologists, sleep specialists, and other healthcare professionals. It's essential to consider the overall clinical picture, including the presence of emotional triggers, associated sleep symptoms, and results from diagnostic tests, to distinguish cataplexy from other conditions with similar presentations.

Treatment Options

The management of cataplexy often involves a combination of lifestyle adjustments, behavioral strategies, and medications. Here are some treatment options for cataplexy:

1. Modifications to Lifestyle:

Establishing Regular Sleep Patterns: Maintaining a consistent sleep schedule, including adequate nighttime sleep and planned daytime naps, can help manage excessive daytime sleepiness associated with cataplexy.

Stress Management: Stress reduction techniques, such as mindfulness, relaxation exercises, and stress management strategies, may help minimize emotional triggers for cataplexy.

Scheduled Naps: Short daytime naps strategically planned to combat sleepiness can be beneficial. However, timing and duration should be discussed with a healthcare professional.

2. Substances:

Selective Serotonin and Norepinephrine Reuptake Inhibitors (SSNRIs): Medications like venlafaxine or duloxetine are often used to manage cataplexy. These drugs help regulate neurotransmitters involved in emotional responses.

Sodium Oxybate: This medication, also known as gamma-hydroxybutyrate (GHB), is a central nervous system depressant that can improve both cataplexy and nighttime sleep in individuals with narcolepsy.

Tricyclic Antidepressants: Medications such as clomipramine or imipramine may be prescribed to reduce the frequency and severity of cataplectic episodes.

3. Orexin Replacement Therapy (Investigational):

Research is ongoing in the development of medications that directly replace or increase the levels of orexin in the brain, addressing the underlying deficiency associated with cataplexy.

4. Counseling and Support:

Psychotherapy: Counseling or psychotherapy may help individuals with cataplexy cope with the emotional and social aspects of living with the condition.

Support Groups: Joining support groups or connecting with others who have narcolepsy and cataplexy can provide valuable insights, shared experiences, and emotional support.

5. Regular Follow-up and Adjustments:

Regular follow-up with healthcare professionals is crucial to monitor the effectiveness of treatment and make any necessary adjustments.

CHAPTER THREE

Treatment approaches may vary based on the individual's specific symptoms, overall health, and response to interventions. A multidisciplinary approach involving neurologists, sleep specialists, and other healthcare professionals can provide comprehensive care for individuals with cataplexy.

Coping Strategies

Living with cataplexy presents unique challenges, but there are coping strategies that individuals can employ to manage its impact on daily life:

1. Knowledge and comprehension:

Learn about cataplexy and its triggers. Understanding the condition can empower individuals to anticipate and manage episodes more effectively.

2. Lifestyle Adjustments:

Establish a consistent sleep schedule to manage excessive daytime sleepiness.

Prioritize stress management techniques, such as mindfulness or relaxation exercises.

3. Emotional Awareness:

Identify and be aware of emotional triggers for cataplexy. Recognizing situations that may lead to episodes allows for proactive coping.

4. Helping Mechanism:

Build a strong support network of friends, family, and healthcare professionals who understand cataplexy and can provide emotional support.

5. Communication:

Communicate openly with friends, family, and colleagues about cataplexy. Educate them on the condition to foster understanding and support.

6. Safety Precautions:

Consider safety measures in environments where episodes may pose a risk. For example, avoid standing near sharp objects during episodes.

7. Medication Management:

Adhere to prescribed medications and communicate regularly with healthcare professionals about their effectiveness and any side effects.

8. Scheduled Naps:

Plan short daytime naps to help manage sleepiness and reduce the likelihood of cataplexy episodes.

9. Stress Reduction Activities:

Engage in activities that promote relaxation and stress reduction, such as yoga, meditation, or hobbies.

10. Counseling and Support Groups:

Consider counseling or joining support groups to address the emotional and social aspects of living with cataplexy.

11. Humor and Positive Outlook:

Maintain a positive outlook and find humor in challenging situations. A positive mindset can contribute to overall well-being.

12. Regular Check-ins with Healthcare Professionals:

Schedule regular follow-up appointments with healthcare professionals to discuss treatment effectiveness and make any necessary adjustments.

Coping with cataplexy involves a combination of self-management strategies, a supportive environment, and ongoing communication with healthcare providers. By proactively addressing the physical and emotional aspects of the condition, individuals with cataplexy can enhance their overall quality of life.

Lifestyle Adjustments

Lifestyle adjustments are crucial for managing cataplexy and minimizing its impact on daily life. Here are some practical recommendations:

1. Sleep Hygiene:

Consistent Sleep Schedule: Maintain a regular sleep routine, going to bed and waking up at the same time every day, even on weekends.

Create a Comfortable Sleep Environment: Ensure the bedroom is dark, quiet, and cool. Consider using blackout curtains and white noise machines if needed.

Limit Stimulants: Reduce or eliminate caffeine and nicotine intake, especially in the hours leading up to bedtime.

2. Scheduled Naps:

Strategic Napping: Plan short and strategic daytime naps to combat excessive sleepiness. Consult with healthcare professionals to determine the optimal nap duration and timing.

Napping Environment: Choose a quiet, comfortable, and dimly lit space for napping.

3. Handling Stress:

Mindfulness and Relaxation Techniques: Practice mindfulness, deep breathing exercises, or progressive muscle relaxation to manage stress and anxiety.

Regular Exercise: Engage in regular physical activity, which can help reduce stress and improve overall well-being. However, avoid intense exercise close to bedtime.

4. Emotional Triggers:

Identify Triggers: Recognize specific emotions that commonly trigger cataplexy episodes. Being aware of these triggers can help individuals anticipate and manage episodes.

Modify Environment: Adjust the environment or circumstances to minimize exposure to known triggers when possible.

5. Safety Measures:

Safe Environments: In settings where episodes may pose a safety risk, take precautions to create a safe environment. For example, avoid standing near sharp objects during episodes.

6. Medication Adherence:

Consistent Medication Use: Adhere to prescribed medications as directed by healthcare professionals. Inform them about any side effects or concerns.

7. Communication:

Open Communication: Communicate openly with friends, family, and colleagues about cataplexy. Educate them about the condition to foster understanding and support.

8. Helping Mechanism:

Build a Support Network: Surround yourself with a supportive network of friends, family, and healthcare professionals who understand cataplexy and can offer assistance when needed.

9. Lifestyle Balance:

Balanced Lifestyle: Strive for a balanced lifestyle that includes adequate sleep, regular physical activity, healthy nutrition, and time for relaxation and leisure.

10. Regular Check-ins with Healthcare Professionals:

Ongoing Evaluation: Schedule regular follow-up appointments with healthcare professionals to assess the effectiveness of treatment strategies and make adjustments as needed.

Adopting these lifestyle adjustments can contribute to better management of cataplexy, improved overall well-being, and a more predictable daily routine. It's essential to tailor these adjustments based on individual preferences and consult with healthcare professionals for personalized guidance.

CONCLUSION

In conclusion, cataplexy is a distinctive and complex neurological phenomenon, often associated with narcolepsy. Characterized by sudden and temporary loss of muscle tone, it poses unique challenges to those affected. The key neurobiological factor is a deficiency in the neurotransmitter orexin, disrupting the delicate balance of the sleep-wake cycle.

Diagnosis involves a thorough clinical assessment, sleep studies, and differentiation from other conditions with similar symptoms. Understanding emotional triggers, such as laughter or excitement, is crucial in managing and coping with cataplexy.

Treatment strategies encompass lifestyle adjustments, medications, and a multidisciplinary approach to address both the physical and emotional aspects. Lifestyle modifications include maintaining a regular sleep schedule, strategic napping, stress management, and creating a supportive environment.

Coping with cataplexy requires a proactive and adaptive mindset. Education, communication with healthcare professionals, and building a strong support network contribute to effective management. By combining these strategies, individuals with cataplexy can enhance their quality of life and navigate the unique challenges associated with this intriguing neurological condition.

THE END

www.ingramcontent.com/pod-product-compliance
Lightning Source LLC
Chambersburg PA
CBHW060844260726
48661CB00002B/590